# The 7-Day Ketogenic

## 35 Delicious
## Low Carb Recipes
## For Weight Loss Motivation

## Volume 1

By

Rachel Richards

First Edition

ISBN-13: 978-0993941511
ISBN-10: 0993941516

# Disclaimer

Disclaimer and Terms of Use: Every effort has been made to ensure that the information in this book is accurate and complete. However, the author and the publisher do not warrant the accuracy of the information, text and graphics contained within the book due to the rapidly changing nature of science, research, known and unknown facts and the internet. The author and the publisher do not hold any responsibility for errors, omissions or contrary interpretation of the subject matter herein. This book is presented solely for motivational and informational purposes only.

Nutritional values have been calculated with due care and attention. However, there may be differences in the calorie count due to the variance of each individual kitchen creation caused by ingredient amounts, brand differences, different cuts and quality of meats etc. The nutritional values of these recipes are provided as a guideline only.

# Table of Contents

# Introduction

### What is the Ketogenic Diet?

Your body uses what you eat to give you energy. Carbohydrates raise your blood sugar levels, and your body reacts by producing insulin to deal with it. Unfortunately, insulin aids in converting glucose to fat, which is then stored in your body's cells.

When following the Ketogenic Diet, it is best to keep your carbohydrate level to below 60g, and preferably around the 20g to 40g level. Slight overage once in a while is not too bad, but where possible less than 50g is the best way to go. This keeps the body in a state of ketosis, whereby the body is burning fat to give a steady stream of energy.

Moderate to high levels of protein and fats are also vital ingredients in ketosis with the fat providing fuel to burn for adequate energy levels. Whilst the actual dietary ingredients of ketosis are important, sensible exercise also plays a big part in losing weight and fine tuning the body's metabolism.

It is essential that you consult your doctor or health professional before embarking on any radical changes in your diet, particularly if you have a lifestyle illness such as diabetes, IBS or any other disease that may be affected by a change in diet.

Most participants of this diet do find that it changes their lives for the good, and creating tasty recipes is a good way to keep their plan in check.

In terms of beverages, drink as much water as possible, but you are also allowed green tea or black coffee. Avoid fizzy drinks, limit alcohol (one drink is fine) and no fruit juices.

The menu recipes are designed for up to 4 people. Every person has a different level of carbohydrate tolerance and participates in a different level of daily exercise. To truly work with a ketogenic diet, you must find your level of carbohydrate tolerance, so a little trial and error or experimentation may be needed. You may mix and match the meal recipes in this book. The 7-day meal plan is merely an example.

If you are trying to lose weight, calorie intake is also important. For men, a daily intake of below 2,000 calories is acceptable. For women, the daily intake is around 1,600 calories. It is difficult to estimate the level of calories for children, as they do expend energy at school and play times, and their metabolism tends to be much faster. It may be necessary for you as an individual to take smaller portions of certain recipes in order to keep your calorie intake at a sensible level.

# Shopping List

This shopping list is designed to help you stay on track during your 7-day plan. Rather than shop every day for the ingredients, we have listed all your store cupboard items together, so that you can purchase these in one visit. The other ingredients are listed per day. Where possible, we have tried to make sure that all goods are used, with little top ups on the necessary days.

## Dried Herbs and Spices, Condiments

- Rosemary, thyme, Italian seasoning, Herbes de Provence, chilli powder, curry powder, Cajun seasoning, mustard seeds, caraway seeds, onion powder, ground coriander
- Black peppercorns, Himalayan salt, garlic powder, star anise powder, yellow mustard, mayonnaise, horseradish sauce, sweet chilli sauce, Tabasco, reduced sugar ketchup, distilled white wine vinegar, dried parmesan

## Baking Products

- Oils – coconut, extra virgin olive oil
- Flours – almond, coconut
- Baking soda
- Vanilla extract, lemon extract, almond extract
- Sweeteners - liquid Stevia, powdered sugar, granulated sugar substitute
- Small bottle of pure or low sugar hazelnut syrup
- Peanut butter
- Coconut flakes
- Pine nuts
- Hazelnuts, chopped or almond slivers
- Ground almonds
- Raw honey

- Unsweetened cocoa powder
- Dark chocolate (high percentage cocoa solids, 75% or more)
- Coffee (your usual brand is fine)
- Small tub of chocolate protein powder
- Ground flaxseed or flaxseed meal
- Chia seeds

## Canned or Jarred Goods/Cartons

- Good quality vegetable stock cubes or powder (you can of course buy ready-made stock, but once opened, must be refrigerated, or make your own vegetable stock)
- Black pitted olives (smallest can available)
- Tuna in spring water (8oz/225g)
- Canned chopped tomatoes (2 x 8oz/225g)
- Small can of tomato puree
- Coconut cream (1 x 8fl oz/240ml) (refrigerate once opened)

## Daily Fresh Purchases (or combine 2 days for ease of shopping)

## Day 1

- 10 eggs (save some for later in the week)
- 8oz/225g chorizo
- 8oz/450g skinless, boneless chicken breasts (for the wraps)
- 4 x 5oz/140g skinless boneless chicken breasts (for the citrus chicken)
- 2 green bell peppers
- 1 large iceberg lettuce
- Small bunch of radishes
- 4 lemons
- 1 lime
- 1 small red onion

- 2 small tomatoes
- ½ cucumber
- Small bunch of rosemary

## Day 2

- 8 fresh eggs
- 8oz/425g butter (you will already have some in the fridge, but top up)
- 16 young baby asparagus spears
- Small bunch fresh mint or parsley
- ½ cucumber (you already have half in the fridge)
- 4oz/115g green beans
- 5oz/140g cauliflower (a small one, or large one cut in half – you will use the rest later in the week)
- 1 medium sized onion
- 1 head of celery (you can use the rest later in the week)
- Small quantity (approximately 4oz/115g baby spinach leaves)
- 3oz/85g mushrooms
- 8oz/225g cream cheese
- 8fl oz/225ml single cream
- 4fl oz/115ml heavy cream or double cream
- 8oz/225g butter (you will not need all of this, but can be used later in the week)
- 14oz/400g mixed crab meat
- 8 x 3½ oz/100g minute steaks
- ¼ bottle red wine

## Day 3

- 12 eggs (some for later in the week)
- 10oz/280g cooked ham from the deli
- 12oz/325g good quality minced pork
- 8oz/225g gruyere cheese
- 8oz/225g mature cheddar cheese
- 4oz/115g cream cheese

- 4oz/115g feta cheese
- 10oz/280g mascarpone cheese
- 8fl oz/240ml half fat milk
- Small bunch scallions/spring onions
- 1 whole garlic bulb (some for later in the week)
- 1 small red chilli
- 1 small knob fresh ginger
- 1 white onion
- 1 carrot (garnish)
- 1lb/425g broccoli
- 1 small bunch chives
- Small bunch of fresh spinach
- Small tub of thick cream
- Small block of butter

## Day 4

- 6 eggs
- 2 large green bell peppers
- 8oz/225g mixed mushrooms, such as shitake, chestnut, button
- 8 Portobello mushrooms
- Small bunch watercress
- Small bunch parsley
- 4oz/115g cheddar cheese
- 40z/115g parmesan cheese
- 1 x goats cheese log (approximately 9oz/250g)
- 8 strawberries (if you like them)
- 1 large savoy cabbage or other crispy cabbage
- 8 lamb steaks (approximately 4oz/115g per steak)

## Day 5

- 8fl oz/240ml half fat milk
- 8fl oz/240ml heavy cream
- 2 ¼ lb/1kg trimmed baby back ribs
- 12oz/325g good quality sausage meat

- 8 strips bacon
- 1 medium sized white cabbage
- 1 carrot
- Small bunch sage
- 8 tender stem broccoli pieces
- 2 ripe avocados
- 1 small red chilli
- 1 small cauliflower
- 1 head of celery
- 1 medium sized red pepper, 1 medium sized green pepper
- 1 small bunch fresh mint
- ½ medium sized cucumber
- 5 medium sized zucchini/courgette

# Day 6

- 6 eggs
- 4oz/115g heavy cream (check to see what you have left)
- 4oz/115g baby spinach (you may still have some left if it is still fresh)
- 3 firm avocados
- 2 tomatoes
- ½ iceberg lettuce
- Small bunch fresh coriander
- Small stalk of lemongrass
- 2 limes
- 1½ lbs/675g mixed greens or your choice
- 1 red onion (you may have one left)
- 3oz/85g hard cheese (check if you have any left)
- 16 medium sized slices of pepperoni
- 1lb/450g ground beef
- 4 slices bacon
- 4 x 5oz/140g boneless salmon fillets

# Day 7

- 10 eggs (check to see how many you have left)
- 1lb/425g good quality sausage meat
- 8 slices deli ham (approximately 8oz/225g)
- 6oz/170g chorizo
- 6oz/170g small cooked prawns
- 8oz/225g cheddar cheese (adjust this if you have some left)
- 8oz/225g heavy or double cream
- 3oz/85g cream cheese
- 4 strips bacon
- 1½ lb/675g cauliflower
- 4 x 6oz/170g sea bass fillets
- 2 head bok choi/pak choi
- 1 small red chilli (you may have some left)
- 1 lime
- ¾in/2cm piece of fresh ginger

# Bonus

As a gift for purchasing this book, you can get an additional recipe, a free printable meal plan and shopping list by visiting the link below:

http://gotorecipecookbooks.com/ketogenic-diet-1/

If you enjoyed the recipes in this book, please take a moment to leave a review.

Thank you for trying out this meal plan book.

For other books by Rachel Richards, visit the website at:

http://RachelRichardsRecipeBooks.com

Good luck!

# 7-Day Meal Plan Chart

## 7-day meal plan

| | DAY 1 | DAY 2 | DAY 3 | DAY 4 | DAY 5 | DAY 6 | DAY 7 |
|---|---|---|---|---|---|---|---|
| Breakfast | Mexican Baked Eggs | Poached Eggs and Asparagus with Herb Butter | Ham and Gruyere Crepes | Mushroom and Pepper Scramble | Bacon and Sausage Parcels | Pepperoni and Cheese Slice | Scotch Eggs |
| Snack | Lettuce Chicken Wraps | Crab Pate on Cucumber Rounds | Cheese and Chive Celery Boats | Parmesan Mustard Crisps | Guacamole with Crudites and Prawns | Avocado 'Fries' | Ham and Prawn Roulades |
| Lunch | Tuna Provencale Salad | Cauliflower and French Bean Crustless Quiche | Ham, Spinach and Feta Frittata | Melting Goats' Cheese Stuffed Mushrooms | Celery and Courgette Soup a La Crème | Keto Brunch Burger | Cauliflower and Chorizo Cheese |
| Snack | Peanut Butter Cookies | Coconut Kisses | Cocoa Choccie Cupcakes | Lemon Cheesecake Bites | Chocolate Mousse | Coconut Pudding | Chocolate Brownie Traybake |
| Dinner | Citrus and Herb Chicken | Succulent Beef Olives | Chinese Sweet and Sour Pork Balls | Lamb with Coconut and Mustard Seeds | Glazed Baby Back Ribs with Coleslaw | Spiced Salmon with Stir Fried Greens | Oriental Sea Bass Parcels |
| TOTAL Calories: | 1392 | 1682 | 1468 | 1725 | 1647 | 1407 | 1494 |
| TOTAL Fat: | 92.2 | 124.5 | 141 | 156 | 90.9 | 112.6 | 106.3 |
| TOTAL Protein: | 82.7 | 121.7 | 89 | 106 | 86.1 | 80.6 | 106.2 |
| TOTAL Carbs: | 19 | 20.2 | 31 | 49.5 | 60 | 22.6 | 26.75 |

# Day 1

# Mexican Baked Eggs

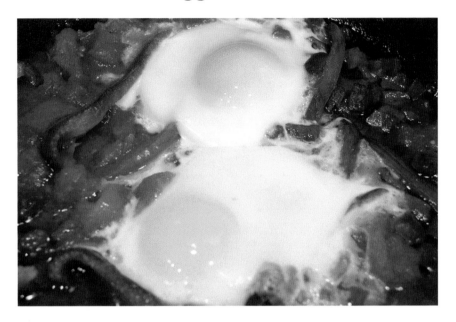

Spicy eggs baked in the oven with peppers and chorizo is an unusual dish with a dash of chilli to add spice. This dish can also be made with pancetta cubes if the chorizo is not to your taste.

**Serves: 4**

**Preparation Time: 5 minutes**

**Cook Time: 10-15 minutes**

Ingredients:

- 2 green bell peppers, core and seeds removed and sliced into strips
- 1 x 8oz/225g chopped canned tomatoes in natural juice
- 8oz/225g chorizo, cubed
- 8 eggs
- Salt and ground pepper to taste
- 2 tsp mild chilli powder

## Method:

1. Heat oven to 180°C/350°F/Gas Mark 4.

2. In an ovenproof large low-sided pan, or 2 pans, similar to a skillet or frying pan, put the chorizo and peppers in over a medium heat. There is no need for oil as the chorizo provides its own oil.

3. Cook until softened, remove from the heat.

4. Crack the eggs separately in cups, to make it easier to place in the pan.

5. Pour in the chopped tomatoes (half into each pan if you are using two) stir in the chilli powder and season.

6. Pour the eggs onto the top of the mix, bake in the oven for 10 minutes. Check to see that the eggs are cooked to your liking.

7. Serve from the oven to the table.

| Nutritional Value | per Portion (2 eggs) |
|---|---|
| Calories | 405 |
| Fat | 33g |
| Carbs | 2.9g |
| Protein | 31g |

# Lettuce Chicken Wraps

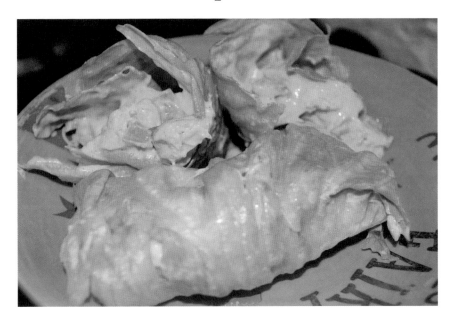

Really easy, and a change from bread wraps or sandwiches, these are wrapped in crisp iceberg lettuce.

**Serves: 4**

**Preparation Time: 10 minutes**

Ingredients:

- 4 small chicken breasts, cooked, or leftover roast chicken (about 8oz/450g)
- 4 large leaves from an iceberg or other crisp lettuce
- 2 tsp mild curry powder
- 2 tbsp mayonnaise
- 2 or 3 radishes, sliced and cut in half

Method:

1. Using either the freshly cooked chicken breasts or the leftover chicken finely shredded or sliced.

2. Mix the chicken, radishes and mayonnaise with the curry powder until combined.

3. Lay out each large lettuce leaf and place a quarter of the mixture on one side, leaving space at either end.

4. Roll up the leaves, tucking the edges in as you go.

5. Serve.

| Nutritional Value | per Portion |
|---|---|
| Calories | 220 |
| Fat | 7g |
| Carbs | 13g |
| Protein | 21g |

# Tuna Provencale Salad

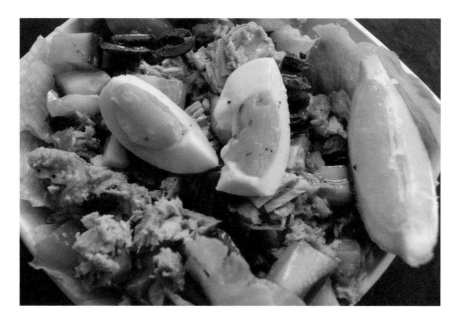

A tasty tuna salad with hints of Provence and packed with healthy protein and fats. Tuna is a classic fish to use on a ketogenic diet, either freshly grilled or from a can – always try to find tuna in spring water, definitely not in brine to keep the sodium content down.

**Serves: 4**

**Preparation Time: 10 minutes**

**Cook Time: 8 minutes (for the hard boiled eggs)**

Ingredients:

- 1lb/425g canned tuna in spring water
- 2 fresh eggs, hard boiled for 8 minutes and shelled, cut into quarters
- Small handful of black pitted olives, chopped (about 8 olives)
- 2 small tomatoes, cut into quarters
- 3 inch/8cm piece of cucumber, diced

- 1 small red onion, cut into thin rings
- 1 cos or iceberg lettuce, washed and broken into pieces
- 3 tbsp olive oil
- Juice of 2 lemons
- Ground black pepper to taste
- 1 tbsp mayonnaise per person, if required

## Method:

1. Drain the tuna and place into a bowl.

2. Break the lettuce into pieces and place in a large salad bowl for serving.

3. Mix in the tomatoes, cucumber and red onion. Set aside.

4. Mix the olive oil with the lemon juice and ground black pepper to taste. Toss into the salad and mix well.

5. Divide the salad between 4 plates, and crumble over the tuna with your fingers.

6. Top with 2 quarters of the hard-boiled egg and sprinkle over the chopped olives.

7. Serve with a tablespoon of mayonnaise per person, if required.

| Nutritional Values | per Portion |
|---|---|
| Calories | 295 |
| Fat | 19.2g |
| Carbs | 9g |
| Protein | 29.1g |

# Peanut Butter Cookies

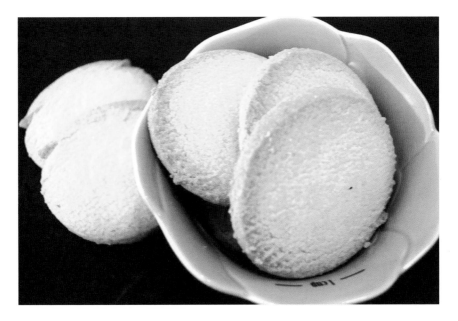

These cookies are delicious for a mid-morning or afternoon snack, or even in a lunchbox for children or adults. Smooth peanut butter is a great addition to a ketogenic diet.

**Serves: 24 medium-sized cookies (serve 2 each, save the rest)**

**Preparation Time: 10 minutes**

**Cook Time: 10-12 minutes**

Ingredients:

- 3½oz/110g smooth peanut butter
- 2oz/55g butter
- 2 large eggs
- 5oz/140g coconut flour
- 5fl.oz/150ml coconut oil
- ½ tsp baking soda
- ½ tsp vanilla extract

- Pinch salt

**Method:**

1. Heat oven to 350°F/180°C/Gas Mark 4.

2. Line 2 flat baking trays with parchment paper.

3. Cream together the peanut butter and butter until combined and fluffy.

4. Add the eggs, coconut oil and vanilla extract and gently mix together until smooth.

5. Above the bowl, sift in the coconut flour, baking soda and pinch of salt and mix until combined with no lumps.

6. Roll into medium sized balls, place on baking sheet and press lightly with a fork to make a round cookie shape. Leave enough space between each as the cookies will spread.

7. Bake for 10-12 minutes until firm and lightly golden.

8. Leave to cool for 5-10 minutes before removing from the parchment paper. Place on a wire rack until completely cool.

Keep remaining cookies from the batch in an airtight container; they will last for up to 5 days.

| Nutritional Values | per portion (2) |
|---|---|
| Calories | 180 |
| Fat | 18g |
| Carbs | 4.1g |
| Protein | 3.6g |

# Citrus and Herb Chicken

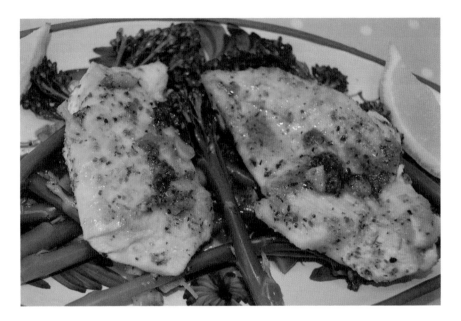

Citrus flavors pair very well with chicken, giving it a delicious tang and zesty taste and aroma. A lovely crisp salad goes well with this dish. Make sure you use the zest of both the lemons and limes; it adds a different dimension to the meal.

**Serves: 4**

**Preparation Time: 10 minutes**

**Cook Time: 20 minutes**

Ingredients:

- 4 x 5oz/140g skinless and boneless chicken breasts
- 4 or 5 tbsp olive oil
- 2 cloves garlic, finely chopped
- Juice and zest of 2 lemons
- Juice and zest of 1 lime
- Freshly ground black pepper

- 2 stalks fresh rosemary, leaves removed and finely chopped

**Method:**

1. Using a fine grater, grate the zest from the lemons and lime. Cut the fruit in half and squeeze out all the juice. Place in a large bowl.

2. Lightly beat the chicken breasts between 2 pieces of cling film.

3. Put the chicken into the bowl with the citrus fruit.

4. Grind over black pepper and mix so that all the chicken is covered.

5. Heat the olive oil in a large skillet over a low to medium heat.

6. Put the chopped garlic into the pan and gently fry, but do not brown.

7. Place the chicken fillets into the pan and continue to fry for 3 or 4 minutes on each side, until lightly browned and cooked through.

8. Pour over the citrus marinade, add the rosemary, turn down the heat and leave to warm through.

9. Serve with a crisp green salad or steamed broccoli.

| Nutritional Values | per Portion |
|---|---|
| Calories | 292 |
| Fat | 23g |
| Carbs | 1.9g |
| Protein | 23g |

# Day 2

# Poached Eggs and Asparagus with Herb Butter

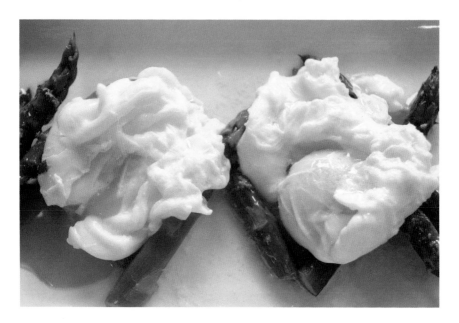

Poached eggs and asparagus have been long term partners, and are a perfect match and a delicious way to start the day.

**Serves: 4**

**Preparation Time: 10 minutes**

**Cook Time: 10 minutes**

Ingredients:

- 16 young asparagus spears
- 8 large eggs
- 5 oz butter
- 2 tbsp fresh parsley or mint, finely chopped
- 3-4oz parmesan, grated

Method:

1.  Snap off the 'woody' ends of the asparagus, if there are any. Place in lightly salted water, bring to the bowl, and leave on a gentle boil for 6-7 minutes until tender, but still al dente. Alternatively you can fry the asparagus in a griddle pan with a mixture of olive oil and butter for the same amount of time.

2.  Crack the eggs into individual cups, if you can, it makes them easier to handle and to form when poured into the pan.

3.  Bring a large pan of water to the boil, stir vigorously in a circular motion and drop each egg into the water.

4.  As there are so many eggs at a time, have a bowl of iced water by the side of the cooker and when the eggs are formed, drop them into the iced water, until each one is finished. When you are ready to serve them, pop back into the hot water to heat through – they will not continue cooking.

5.  In the meantime, melt the butter, add the herbs and stir until ready.

6.  Lay out the asparagus spears on each plate, top with the warmed poached eggs and pour over the herby butter.

7.  A little grated parmesan over the top is also a delicious addition to this dish.

| Nutritional Value | per Portion |
|---|---|
| Calories | 583 |
| Fat | 50g |
| Carbs | 1g |
| Protein | 31g |

# Crab Pate on Cucumber Rounds

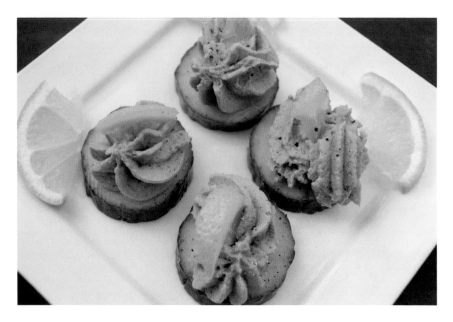

Crab pate is mouth-wateringly delicious at any time of the day, and whilst it is usual to use Melba toast, we have used rounds of cucumber as the substitute for bread. Easy to make, can be used for a snack or a starter for a dinner party.

**Serves: 4 (16 rounds – 4 per person)**

**Preparation Time: 10 minutes**

**Cook Time: Not required**

Ingredients:

- 14oz/400g mixed crab meat
- 7oz/200g cream cheese, such as Philadelphia
- 2 heaped tsp horseradish sauce
- 1 tbsp mayonnaise
- Freshly ground black pepper
- Juice of half a lemon
- 1 lemon, cut into small thin triangles

- 1 cucumber, cut into ½ inch/1cm rounds

**Method:**

1. In a medium sized bowl, mix all the ingredients together, except the cucumber. Season to taste.

2. If you don't like the skin, peel the cucumber before slicing into rounds, otherwise leave intact. You should be able to get 16 rounds out of a medium sized cucumber.

3. Using a teaspoon, heap 2 tsp of the crab mixture on to each cucumber round. Season with more black pepper and add a small piece of lemon on the top for decoration, or squeezing over the crab.

| Nutritional Value | per Portion |
|---|---|
| Calories | 306 |
| Fat | 21g |
| Carbs | 6g |
| Protein | 26g |

# Cauliflower and French Bean Crustless Quiche

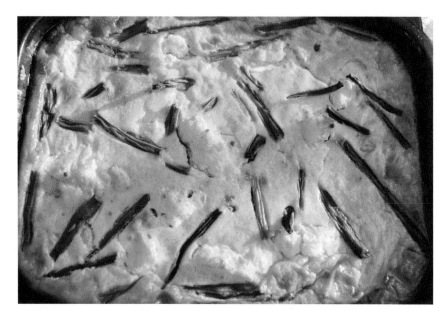

This is a very tasty quiche when made with lots of strong cheese or blue cheese. We have used very strong cheddar cheese, but you can use a salty blue cheese. If you use blue cheese, be careful with the amount of salt seasoning you may add – the saltiness of the cheese increases during the cooking period. You can use a smaller but slightly deeper dish for this, such as a small non-stick roaster.

**Serves: 4**

**Preparation Time: 20 minutes**

**Cook Time: 20-25 minutes**

Ingredients:

- 5oz/140g cauliflower, broken into small florets
- 4oz/115g green beans, cut into 1½inch/3cm pieces
- 4 eggs

- 225ml/8fl.oz single cream, or half cream and half yoghurt
- Seasoning to taste (easy on the salt if using blue cheese), but extra pepper
- 4oz/115g of strong cheddar cheese, grated (try to get a coloured cheddar)
- 1 tsp of dried Herbes de Provence

Method:

1. Heat the oven to 180°C/350°F/Gas mark 4.

2. While the oven is heating, cook the cauliflower florets and green beans for approximately 10 minutes until just tender. Drain until dry.

3. Mix together the eggs, cream and herbs. Add half of the grated cheese and mix well. Season.

4. Pour half the egg mixture into your dish and then the vegetables, evenly distributed. Top up with the remaining egg mixture, and sprinkle over the last of the grated cheese. Place on a baking tray.

5. Bake in the oven for 20 minutes and test the middle of the quiche. If a knife comes out clean and the mix is firm to the touch, remove from the oven. If not, bake for a further 5 minutes.

6. Serve with a green salad or cumin spiced roasted vegetables.

| Nutritional Values | per Portion |
|---|---|
| Calories | 225 |
| Fat | 19.5g |
| Carbs | 4g |
| Protein | 13.2g |

# Coconut Kisses

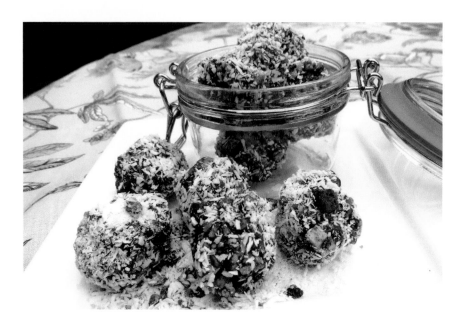

A little bit of fun and indulgence, these little coconut and chocolate balls are great for a coffee break or an afternoon snack when you are craving a little bit of sweetness.

**Serves: 16 medium sized 'kisses' (2 per person, save the rest)**

**Preparation Time: 20 minutes**

**Cooling Time: 30 minutes (should be kept in the refrigerator)**

Ingredients:

- 4fl.oz/120ml double or heavy cream
- 4oz/115g dark chocolate (90% cocoa solids), chopped into small pieces
- 12oz/325g almond flour (a little extra if needed)
- 2oz/55g butter
- 1 tsp vanilla extract
- 4-5oz/115-140g coconut flakes

Method:

1. Place the cream in a small pan over a low heat, add the chocolate and stir until melted together.

2. Add the butter and stir until the mixture has thickened.

3. Stir in the almond flour and vanilla essence until everything is combined and not lumps. The mixture should be very thick and fudgy.

4. Dust a preparation board with a thick layer of coconut flakes.

5. When cool, divide the mixture into 16 separate balls.

6. Roll each ball in the coconut until completely covered.

7. Refrigerate until firm, and serve when you are ready to eat them!

Save the rest for guests – or substitute one of the snacks later in the week if you fall in love with them!

| Nutritional Value | per Portion (2 each) |
|---|---|
| Calories | 172 |
| Fat | 14.8 |
| Carbs | 7.1 |
| Protein | 3.5g |

# Succulent Beef Olives

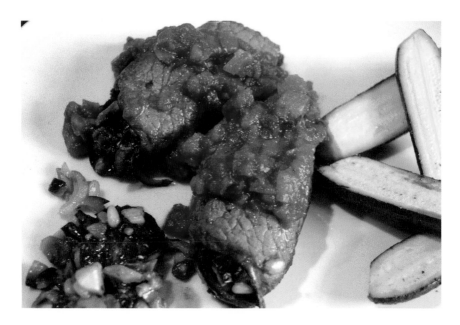

Beef olives (there are no olives in this dish, in spite of the name!) braised in a red wine and tomato stock are truly delicious. You can vary the stuffing of the beef with other ingredients that you may like, but this one works really well.

**Serves: 4**

**Preparation Time: 10 minutes**

**Cook Time: 1 hour**

Ingredients:

- 8 x 100g/3½oz slices of lean beef (minute steaks are a good choice)
- 2 tbsp strong mustard
- 1 medium onion, finely chopped
- 8 mushrooms, finely chopped
- 2 sticks of celery, finely chopped
- 2 garlic cloves, finely chopped

- 2 tbsp olive oil
- Small handful baby spinach leaves
- 2oz/55g pine nuts

For the sauce

- 600ml/20fl.oz beef stock
- 3 tbsp tomato puree or passata
- 150ml/5fl.oz red wine
- 2 tbsp rosemary, leaves only, chopped

Method:

1. Heat oven to 180°C/350°F/Gas Mark 4. Lightly 'bash' out each piece of beef so that they are about 6 millimetres/¼ inch thick. Brush each piece with mustard.

2. In a pan, gently fry off the onions, mushrooms, garlic and celery until soft.

3. Add the spinach and pine nuts and stir together.

4. Starting at one edge, divide the filling between each of the slices, and roll tightly to a cylinder. Use cocktail sticks to keep the roll together. Place in a baking dish.

5. Mix the red wine and stock in a pan and bring to the boil, then simmer for 5 minutes.

6. Add the tomato puree/passata and the rosemary and simmer for a further 5 minutes.

7. Pour the sauce over/ the beef, and cook in the oven for 45 minutes – 1 hour, covered in foil to prevent burning.

8. Serve with fresh seasonal non-root vegetables.

| Nutritional Values | per Portion |
|---|---|
| Calories | 396 |
| Fat | 19.2 |
| Carbs | 2.1 |
| Protein | 48g |

# Day 3

# Ham and Gruyere Crepes

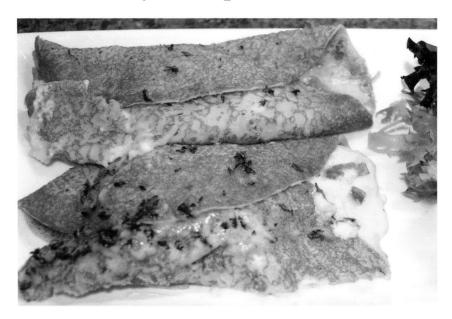

A very quick and tasty dish, suitable for brunch, light lunch or supper. You can substitute the all-purpose flour for buckwheat flour, which gives a nuttier taste, and a more authentic taste of France where these tasty morsels originate from.

**Serves: Approximately 4-5 crepes**

**Prep Time: 10 minutes**

**Cook Time: 15-20 mins**

Ingredients:

- 8fl.oz/240ml half fat milk
- 1 egg
- 2½oz/70g almond flour
- ½ tsp olive oil
- 8 tsp unsalted butter
- ½ tsp salt
- 10oz/280g cooked ham, shredded

- 8oz/225g Gruyere cheese, grated
- Ground pepper to taste
- 2 tbsp fresh chives, finely chopped

**Method:**

1. Heat oven to 170°C/325°F/Gas mark 3.

2. Beat the milk, eggs, olive oil and flour together, add the salt and beat again until smooth and runny. Refrigerate for one hour if possible, or overnight.

3. Heat a frying pan or crepe pan (if you have one) with a little of the butter, to coat the bottom of the pan.

4. Pour 2 large tbsp of batter into the pan; swirl around to coat (off the heat). Replace on to the heat and cook for 1-2 minutes until the underside of the crepe is cooked. Flip over with a spatula, and cook the other side until lightly brown.

5. Remove from the pan and place on to baking paper. Repeat the process until you have enough crepes, putting a piece of baking paper between each one and ensuring you re-grease the pan.

6. On a clean board, assemble the crepes, with the shredded ham, gruyere and a few sprinkles of the chives. Fold the pancakes over and place in a baking dish.

7. Bake for about 8 minutes, or until the cheese has melted and the filling is hot.

8. Serve with a tossed green salad and vinaigrette.

| Nutritional Value | per Portion (1 crepe) |
|---|---|
| Calories | 230 |
| Fat | 16g |
| Carbs | 8.9g |
| Protein | 21g |

# Cheese and Chive Celery Boats

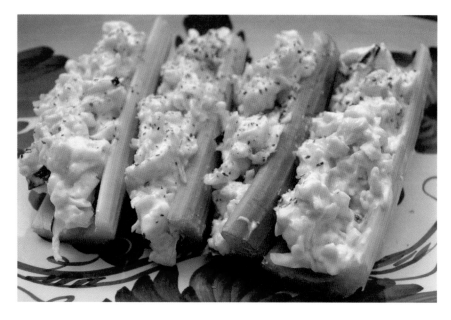

Delicious crunchy snack, or if cut smaller, a lovely canapé for a party. We have used a strong cheddar, but you can use blue cheese if you prefer, or possibly a soft cheese such as ripe brie or camembert.

**Serves: 4**

**Preparation Time: 15-20 minutes**

**Cook Time: No Cooking Required**

Ingredients:

- 8 medium sized celery sticks, cut in half or in three
- 2 heaped tbsp soft cream cheese
- 4oz/115g cheddar cheese, grated
- 2 tbsp mayonnaise
- 4 chives, finely chopped
- ½ tsp cayenne or paprika, to sprinkle over

Method:

1. Wash and strip the celery of and stringy bits and then cut into portions.

2. Mix together the cream cheese, cheddar, mayonnaise and chives.

3. Fill each celery 'boat' with the mixture and sprinkle over the paprika/cayenne.

4. Serve.

| Nutritional Value | per Portion (2 or 3 sticks depending how cut) |
|---|---|
| Calories | 139 |
| Fat | 15g |
| Carbs | Trace |
| Protein | 1g |

# Ham, Spinach and Feta Frittata

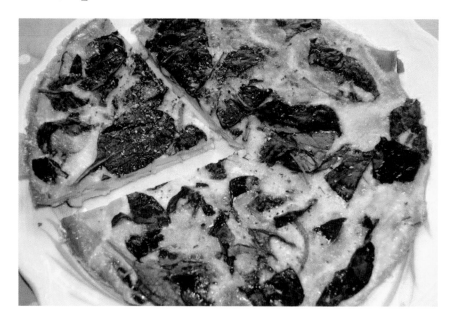

Make this dish in one big frying pan or skillet, and simply cut into wedges to serve. Serve with a leafy green salad and cucumber for a filling lunch. Very simple to make.

**Serves: 4**

**Preparation Time: 5 minutes**

**Cook Time: 15 minutes**

Ingredients:

- 10 eggs, beaten
- 6 slices deli ham (about 4oz/115g) chopped or sliced into ribbons
- 2 tbsp thick cream
- 2 large handfuls of baby spinach
- 4oz/115g feta cheese, finely crumbled
- 2 cloves garlic, minced
- Freshly ground black pepper, to taste

- 1 tsp dried mixed herbs, or Herbes de Provence
- 2 tbsp butter

Method:

1. Heat grill. Make sure you have enough space on the second shelf under the grill (if in the oven), or the bottom of the grill (take out any shelves).

2. Mix together the eggs and cream. Add pepper to taste. Mix in the minced garlic, herbs and feta cheese.

3. In a large frying pan or skillet, melt the butter on the top of the stove until gently foaming. Pour in the most of the egg mixture, scatter over the ham and the spinach. Top with remaining egg mixture.

4. Leave on the top of the oven for a couple of minutes until the bottom appears to be set.

5. Place under the grill and cook until set.

6. Cut into slices and serve.

| Nutritional Values | per Portion |
|---|---|
| Calories | 456 |
| Fat | 38g |
| Carbs | 1g |
| Protein | 28g |

# Cocoa Choccie Cupcakes

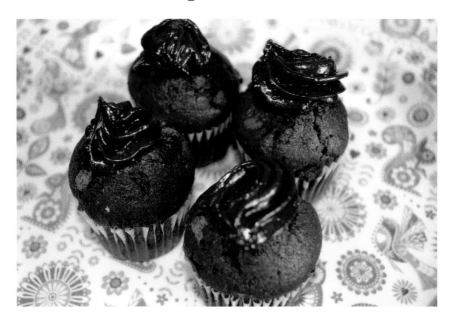

A good treat for an afternoon snack or at morning coffee time. Perfect for a ketogenic diet, with good amounts of fat and protein, and extremely low carbs.

**Serves: 4 (makes 12 cupcakes, portion based on 1 per person, so store the rest in airtight container)**

**Preparation Time: 10 minutes**

**Cook Time: 15-20 minutes**

Ingredients:

- 10oz/280g mascarpone cheese
- 1oz/30g ground almonds
- 2 fresh eggs, separated
- 4 scoops (scoop is provided in container) chocolate protein powder
- 1oz/30g cocoa powder (unsweetened)

- 2fl.oz/60ml strongly flavored coffee (you could use some left over from coffee machine)
- 1 tsp liquid stevia or similar sugar substitute
- ½ tsp vanilla essence

Method:

1. Heat the oven to 170°C/325°F/Gas Mark 3.

2. Prepare a lightly greased cupcake tin (use butter for greasing) or use cupcake cases placed on a baking tray.

3. Mix half of the chocolate protein powder with the ground almonds and cocoa.

4. Beat the egg whites until stiff but fluffy. Fold the egg whites into the dry mixture.

5. In a different bowl, loosen half of the mascarpone and gently fold into the mixture. Pour evenly into each cupcake receptacle, or into each cupcake case.

6. Place the cupcake tray into the oven and bake for 15 minutes – check if cooked by inserting a skewer into the centre, and if it comes out clean, remove from oven. Otherwise, continue to cook for a few more minutes until firm.

7. Whilst the cupcakes are cooking, mix together the egg yolks, the remaining chocolate protein powder, mascarpone, stevia and vanilla essence (this is for a delicious icing).

8. Remove cakes from the oven, leave to cool.

9. With the ready-made or leftover coffee, pour this over each cake to soak in. When completely cool, top with the icing.

10. Please note that protein powders vary between manufacturers – we have based this upon 1 scoop of powder (supplied with the product) being 20g.

Save remaining cakes in an airtight container in the fridge. They will keep for up to 5 days.

| Nutritional Values | per Portion (1 cake) |
|---|---|
| Calories | 106 |
| Fat | 10g |
| Carbs | 1g |
| Protein | 3g |

# Chinese Sweet and Sour Pork Balls

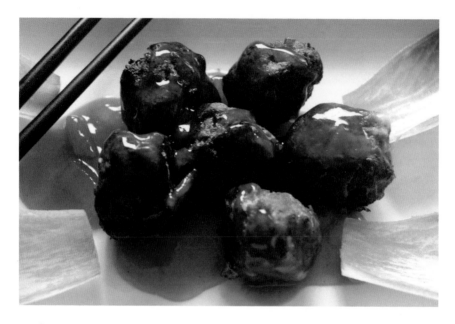

This is a very filling and extremely yummy dish which everyone will love, particularly the children.

**Serves: 4 (20 balls)**

**Preparation Time: 10-15 minutes**

**Cook Time: 20 minutes**

Ingredients:

<u>For the pork balls</u>

- 4oz/115g white onion, minced
- 1lb/450g ground or minced pork
- 1 tbsp butter
- 1 tsp salt
- ½ tsp star anise powder
- 4oz/115g coconut flour
- 1 egg, beaten to bind

- 4oz/115g  hard but mild cheese, grated

For the sweet and sour sauce

- 2 tsp liquid stevia
- 8 tbsp reduced sugar ketchup
- 6fl.oz/180ml distilled white wine vinegar
- 2 tsp garlic powder

Method:

1. Heat oven to 350°F/180°C/Gas mark 4

2. Mix all of the sauce ingredients together in a pan and heat gently. When just coming up to the bowl, turn off the heat.

3. In a large bowl mix together the pork, onions, cheese, star anise, salt and half the flour. Add the beaten egg and combine thoroughly.

4. Mould into balls and roll in the remaining flour.

5. Place on a baking sheet, and bake in the oven for 10 minutes, turn and bake for a further 10 minutes.

6. When cooked, turn off the oven and leave the pork balls in there. Reheat the sauce. When sauce is warmed through, remove pork balls from the oven.

7. Serve on plates with steamed broccoli and some sauce poured over the top.

| Nutritional Value | per Portion |
|---|---|
| Calories | 537 |
| Fat | 27g |
| Carbs | 25g |
| Protein | 49g |

# Day 4

# Mushroom and Pepper Scramble

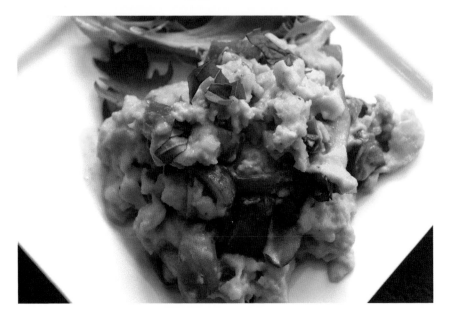

Delicious scrambled eggs, with oodles of mushrooms and crunchy green peppers!

**Serves: 4**

**Preparation Time: 10 minutes**

**Cook Time: 8-10 minutes**

Ingredients:

- 8 oz/225g mushrooms, washed and sliced (a selection of different mushrooms is the best, such as chestnut, shitake and button)
- 1 large green bell pepper, core and seeds removed and diced
- 8 large fresh eggs
- 2 tbsp heavy (double) cream
- 4 tbsp butter
- 3 tsp fresh parsley, finely chopped
- Salt and freshly ground black pepper, to taste

- Handful of watercress to garnish

**Method:**

1. Break the eggs into a jug and whisk until combined.

2. Add the cream and seasoning, whisk again and set aside.

3. Place half of the butter into a frying pan or skillet over a medium heat until foaming.

4. Place the chopped peppers into the pan and gently fry until softened.

5. Add the mushrooms and continue to fry until soft, but not mushy. Remove from the pan and leave to one side.

6. Melt the remaining butter over a low heat and scramble the eggs until a little creamy.

7. Add the mushrooms and peppers back into the pan with the chopped parsley.

8. Continue to cook for a further minute until set but not dry.

9. Serve on warm plates with a little watercress for garnish.

| Nutritional Values | per Portion |
|---|---|
| Calories | 310 |
| Fat | 26g |
| Carbs | 3g |
| Protein | 19g |

# Parmesan Mustard Crisps

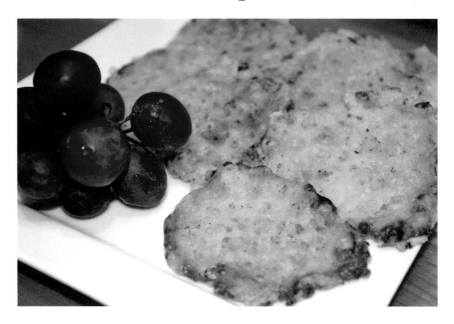

These tasty crunchy morsels will stave off the hunger between meals and have a little bit of a kick to them with the addition of mustard. So simple to make, you will be keeping these as a regular addition to your weekly snacks.

**Serves: 4 (5 crisps per person)**

**Preparation Time: 5 minutes**

**Cook Time: 10-12 minutes**

Ingredients:

- 4oz/115g parmesan cheese, grated
- 4oz/115g cheddar cheese, grated
- 1 tbsp mustard (depending how hot you like it, you can use English mustard or a milder yellow mustard)

Method:

1. Heat oven to 200°C/400°F/Gas Mark 6

2. Place the grated cheese in a bowl and carefully mix in the mustard, so that it spreads through the mixture.

3. Prepare a baking tray by covering with parchment paper.

4. Put small clusters of the cheese mix onto the tray, leaving spaces between each one, as the mixture will spread out quite a lot.

5. Bake in the oven for 10 minutes, or until the mixture is bubbling and going slightly brown round the edges.

6. Remove from the oven and leave to cool before taking the crisps off the parchment.

| Nutritional Values | per Portion |
|---|---|
| Calories | 90 |
| Fat | 6g |
| Carbs | 1g |
| Protein | 8g |

# Melting Goats' Cheese Stuffed Mushrooms

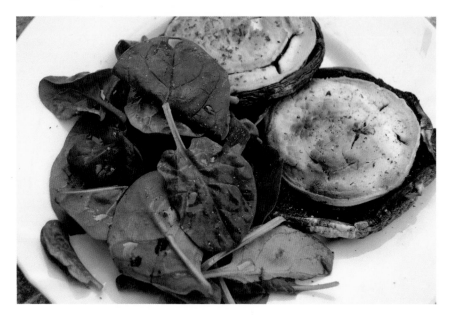

Combining goats' cheese and mushroom is a classical pairing from European food. The mushroom melts in your mouth, and the subtle hint of goats cheese and garlic makes for a tender and delicious experience.

**Serves: 4**

**Preparation Time: 10 minutes**

**Cook Time: 15 minutes**

Ingredients:

- 8 large field or Portobello mushrooms
- 3 cloves garlic, chopped
- 9oz/250g log of goats cheese, sliced into 8 rounds
- 2 tbsp olive oil
- 2 tbsp dried Italian seasoning (mixed herbs)
- 4 slices deli ham, cut into pieces

Method:

1. Heat oven to 200°C/400°F/Gas mark 6

2. Clean the mushrooms and pat dry. Place on a foil lined baking tray, gill side up.

3. Portion the chopped garlic and ham in each of the mushrooms. Top with a round of goats cheese.

4. Drizzle the mushrooms with the oil and scatter over the herbs.

5. Bake in the oven for 10-15 minutes (depending on how big the mushroom is) until the cheese is bubbling.

6. Serve with a watercress salad.

| Nutritional Value | per Portion |
|---|---|
| Calories | 287 |
| Fat | 26g |
| Carbs | 3g |
| Protein | 17g |

# Lemon Cheesecake Bites

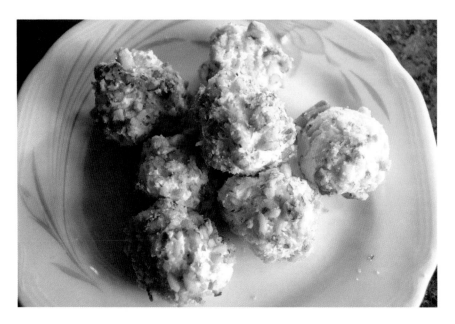

As well as being a little sweet snack, these are quite refreshing as they are not overly sweet and nice and nutty.

**Serves: 4 (16 pieces)**

**Preparation Time: 15 minutes**

**Cook Time: No cooking required**

Ingredients:

- 8oz/225g cream cheese
- 3oz/85g powdered sugar (substitute for icing sugar)
- 2 tbsp double or heavy cream
- 1 or 2 drops (to taste) lemon extract
- ½ tbsp sugar free hazelnut syrup
- 2-3 oz/55-85g chopped hazelnuts (or almonds)
- 8 strawberries (if desired)

Method:

1. Mix the cream cheese, powdered sugar and cream together, beating firmly to combine the mixture.

2. Add the lemon extract and hazelnut syrup (you can use raw honey as a substitute). The mixture should be quite firm, so that you are able to roll into balls. If too loose, add a little more powdered sugar to firm up.

3. With slightly damp hands, roll the mixture into balls in the palms of your hands.

4. Spread out the nuts on a board, and roll each cheesecake ball so that that they are covered in nuts.

5. Place in small paper cases, like truffle or mini muffin cases and refrigerate until ready to eat.

6. Try adding a strawberry or two to eat with them – this is allowed once in a while. You can also spread this mix in a tray with a flat layer of nuts on the bottom and the cheesecake mix on the top, and cut into small squares to eat.

Please note, this recipe is high in calories and carbohydrates. Suggested amount would be 2 per person, depending on exercise rate. Save the rest for guests!

| Nutritional Values | per Portion |
|---|---|
| Calories | 718 (per 4 pieces) |
| Fat | 65g |
| Carbs | 25g |
| Protein | 10g |

# Lamb with Coconut and Mustard Seeds

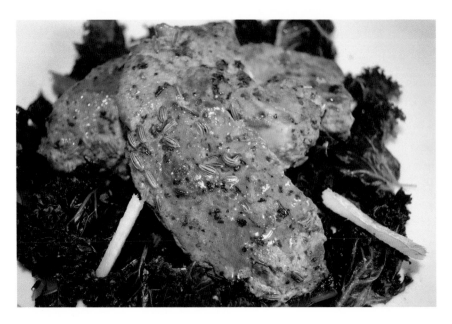

Lovely, juicy lamb Middle Eastern style and served with crisp stir fried cabbage make a quick and delicious meal. You can add more vegetables such as green beans. Serve with a delicious raita (yoghurt, mint and cucumber sauce).

**Serves: 4**

**Preparation Time: 20 minutes**

**Cook Time: 15 minutes**

Ingredients:

- 8-12 lamb steaks or cutlets, depending on size (2 minimum per person)
- 1 tbsp ground coriander
- 3 tbsp black mustard seeds
- 1 thumb-sized piece of ginger, shredded into matchsticks
- 2 cloves garlic, peeled and finely chopped
- 3 tbsp unrefined coconut oil

- 1 large savoy cabbage, or crispy cabbage, shredded
- Grind of black pepper, to season to taste
- Olive oil for frying
- 4 oz/115g Greek Yoghurt
- 1 tbsp fresh mint, chopped finely
- 2in/1cm piece of cucumber, chopped

Method:

1. Prepare all the ingredients as above. Place the coconut oil into a shallow sided bowl and add the mustard seeds, coriander and some black pepper. Add the ginger and garlic and stir thoroughly.

2. Marinate the lamb in the coconut mixture for at least 15 minutes, longer if you have time.

3. Take a griddle pan and fry the cutlets until golden brown but not well done. You could also cook them under a hot grill, approximately 5 minutes each side for nice and juicy pink lamb.

4. Whilst frying the lamb, place the olive oil into another pan and stir fry the crisp cabbage until cooked, but still a little crunchy.

5. Make the mint and yoghurt dip by mixing all the ingredients together in a bowl.

6. Serve the lamb on top of the cabbage with extra vegetables, and let people help themselves to the dip

| Nutritional Value | per Portion |
|---|---|
| Calories | 320 |
| Fat | 25g |
| Carbs | 5.6g |
| Protein | 27g |

# Day 5

# Bacon and Sausage Parcels

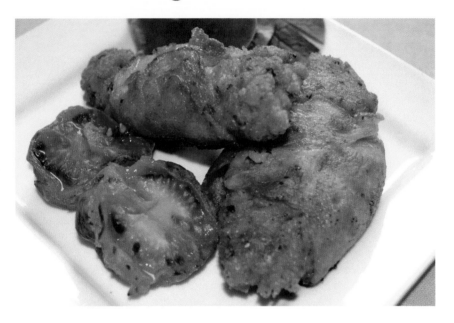

A warm and filling start to the day. The parcels can be prepared the night before and cooked in the morning. Good quality sausage meat with chopped fresh sage is the key to this dish. You could also add chopped peppers or even chilli if you like your life a little spicy!

**Serves: 4 (2 per person)**

**Preparation Time: 10 minutes**

**Cook Time: 15 minutes**

Ingredients:

- 12oz/325g good quality sausage meat
- 3 tsp fresh sage, finely chopped
- 1 tbsp olive oil
- Freshly ground black pepper to season
- 8 strips or rashers of bacon

Method:

1. Heat oven to 180°C/350°F/Gas mark 4

2. In a bowl, combine the sausage meat with the sage and ground black pepper (add peppers or chilli if this is to your taste).

3. Portion the sausage meat into 8, and roll the sausage meat mix in the palm of your hand to form a log shape. Wrap with one slice of bacon.

4. Heat the olive oil over a low heat, and gently seal each of the parcels.

5. Place on a foil lined baking tray and bake in the oven for 10-15 minutes, until the sausage meat is cooked through and the bacon is a light golden brown.

6. In the latter stages of cooking, you can drizzle the parcels with a little honey or maple syrup.

| Nutritional Value | per Portion (2 each) |
|---|---|
| Calories | 395 |
| Fat | 32g |
| Carbs | 9g |
| Protein | 17g |

# Guacamole with Crudites and Prawns

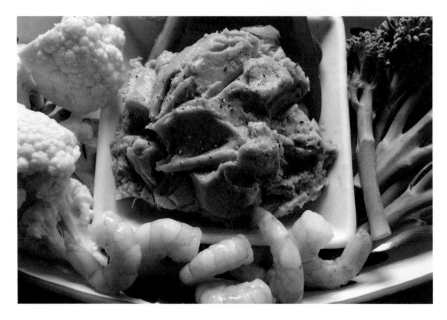

This is a lovely snack to share amongst friends and family. You can add a little spice to the guacamole to bring out the flavor. The crudités can be varied but we have used cauliflower and broccoli with the prawns.

**Serves: 4**

**Preparation Time: 15 minutes**

**Cook Time: No cooking required**

Ingredients:

- 2 ripe avocados, peeled, stoned and mashed
- 1 small red or green chilli, finely chopped
- 1 tsp Tabasco
- 1 small cauliflower, cut into florets
- 8 tender stem broccoli pieces, ends removed
- 1 green pepper, seeds and core removed, sliced
- 4oz/113g prawns or shrimp

**Method:**

1. In a bowl, mix together the avocados, chilli and Tabasco.

2. Place on a serving dish, and display the cauliflower, broccoli and pepper with the prawns, around the dip.

3. Serve.

| Nutritional Value | per Portion |
|---|---|
| Calories | 158 |
| Fat | 12g |
| Carbs | 5g |
| Protein | 8g |

# Celery and Courgette Soup a La Crème

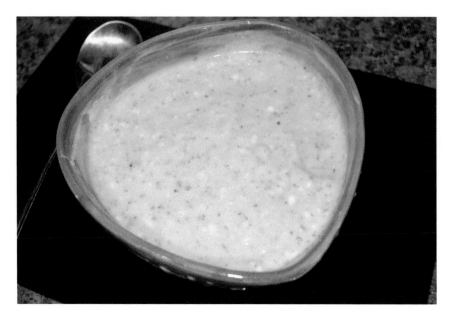

A lovely cream of celery soup that can be served hot or cold depending on the weather.

**Serves: 4**

**Preparation Time: 10-15 minutes**

**Cook Time: 5 minutes if served hot**

Ingredients:

- 5 medium sized zucchini/courgette, unpeeled and diced
- 8 celery stalks, washed, stringy pieces removed and diced
- 1 medium red pepper, core and seeds removed, diced
- 1 medium green pepper, core and seeds removed, diced
- 1 medium sized cucumber, washed, unpeeled and diced
- 4 tbsp extra virgin olive oil
- 8fl.oz/240ml heavy/double cream
- 1½ tbsp fresh mint, chopped

- Salt and pepper to taste

Method:

1. Place all the prepared vegetables in a food processor, juicer or liquidiser.

2. Process until almost smooth, then add the olive oil and cream. Pulse on low until all ingredients are mixed together and smooth.

3. Test for seasoning.

4. If required warm, gently heat for 5 minutes, do not boil.

5. Serve in bowls with a sprinkling of chopped mint on each.

| Nutritional Value | per Portion |
| --- | --- |
| Calories | 285 |
| Fat | 26.2g |
| Carbs | 11.9g |
| Protein | 5.6g |

# Chocolate Mousse

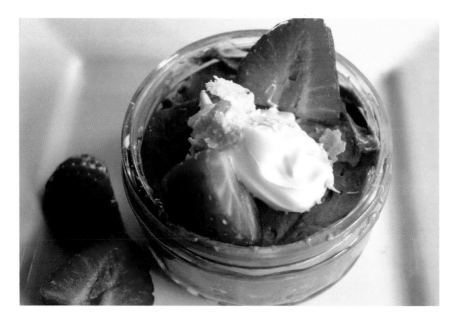

This recipe will solve any sweet attacks you may have! Using dark chocolate with around 80% cocoa butter is ideal. Make the day before and leave in the refrigerator.

**Serves: 4**

**Preparation Time: 10 minutes, plus minimum 1 hour cooling**

**Cook Time: 5 minutes**

Ingredients:

- ½ can coconut cream (must be coconut cream)
- 7 tbsp water
- 6 oz/170g dark chocolate
- ½ tsp almond extract, or vanilla if preferred for sweeter taste

Method:

1. Melt the chocolate and water together over a low heat. Scrape all the mixture into a medium sized bowl.

2.  Beat the mixture with an electric whisk for about 5 minutes, until it becomes soft and 'fluffy'. It needs to hold its shape.

3.  Spoon into small ramekins or dishes (even small glassware). Refrigerate until ready to eat.

4.  Prior to serving, beat the coconut cream and almond or vanilla extract together using an electric whisk, preferably, until the mixture is reasonably firm.

5.  Pipe or put approximately 1 heaped tablespoon of the cream mixture onto the top of the mousse.

6.  Ready to serve.

| Nutritional Value | per Portion |
|-------------------|-------------|
| Calories | 125 |
| Fat | 9.7g |
| Carbs | 9.2g |
| Protein | 2.5g |

# Glazed Baby Back Ribs with Coleslaw

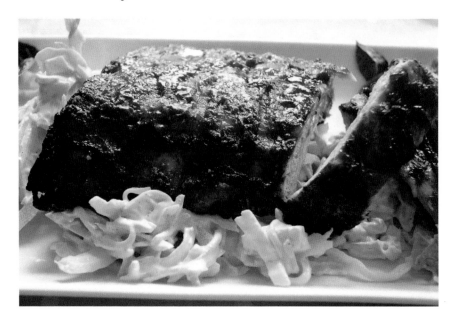

These take a little while to cook, but the result is worthwhile. Freshly made coleslaw is a great accompaniment to these delicious ribs.

**Serves: 4**

**Preparation Time: 15 minutes**

**Cook Time: 1 hr 15 min – 1hr 30 min**

Ingredients:

- 2¼lb/1kg trimmed baby back ribs, cut into 4 separate racks
- 3 tbsp olive oil
- 2 tbsp mild Cajun seasoning
- 2 cloves garlic, crushed
- 1 tbsp raw honey
- 1 medium sized white cabbage, shredded
- 1 medium sized red onion

- ½ small carrot, julienned or cut into matchsticks (you can grate but there is more of a crunch if julienned or cut into sticks)
- 1 tsp mustard seeds
- 1 tsp caraway seeds
- 1½ heaped tbsp mayonnaise

Method:

1. Heat oven to 350°F/180°C/Gas mark 4

2. Mix together the marinade for the ribs by placing the olive oil, Cajun seasoning, raw honey and garlic together in a small bowl. Using a small pastry brush, cover the ribs with the marinade. Keep any remaining marinade to one side.

3. Place the ribs in a shallow baking tray into the oven.

4. Cook for 40 minutes, remove from the oven and baste with the remaining marinade. Cook for a further 40 minutes and test to ensure the ribs are cooked. If not, place back in the oven for a further 10 minutes.

5. Whilst the ribs are cooking, make your coleslaw. In a large bowl, mix together the white cabbage, onion, carrot, mustard seeds and caraway seeds. Spoon in the mayonnaise and mix well. Place in the refrigerator.

6. When the ribs are cooked, remove from the oven, place on a bed of coleslaw and serve.

| Nutritional Value | per Portion |
|-------------------|-------------|
| Calories | 684 |
| Fat | 46g |
| Carbs | 20g |
| Protein | 40g |

# Day 6

# Pepperoni and Cheese Slice

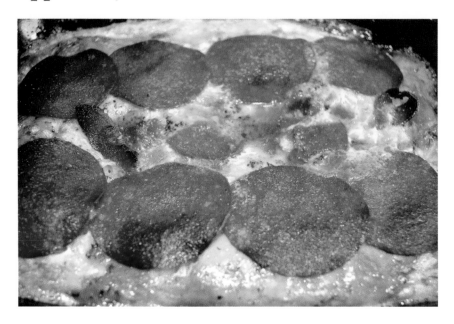

Almost like a crustless pizza, a rectangle of this in the morning for breakfast will give you a good start to the day.

**Serves: 4**

**Preparation Time: 15 minutes**

**Cook Time: 25 minutes**

Ingredients:

- 6 eggs
- 2 handfuls baby spinach
- 16 medium-sized slices pepperoni
- 3oz/85g cheddar cheese, grated
- Olive oil for greasing
- Seasoning to taste (plenty of ground black pepper)

Method:

1. Heat oven to 350°F/180°C/Gas mark 4

2. Lightly oil an 8 x 8in/20 x 20cm roasting or baking tin.

3. Put the spinach in the bottom of the tin. Lay 8 of the pepperoni slices over the top, spaced evenly.

4. Whisk the eggs and add the grated cheese. Stir to combine. Season.

5. Pour the mix over the pepperoni and spinach, then top with the remaining pepperoni.

6. Bake in the oven for 20-25 minutes until firm to the touch.

| Nutritional Value | per Portion |
|---|---|
| Calories | 307 |
| Fat | 24.1g |
| Carbs | 1.1g |
| Protein | 22.8g |

# Avocado 'Fries'

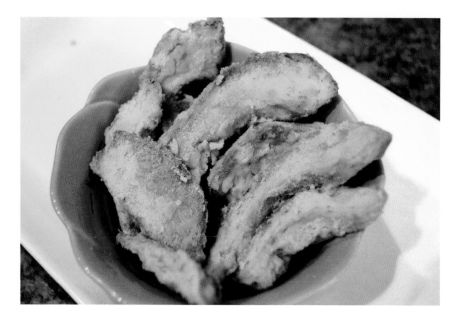

These little guys are absolutely yummy, quite quick to make, and worthwhile as a part of your keto diet. For a really great dinner, you can serve these with your burger as opposed to a snack for a really filling meal.

**Serves: 4**

**Preparation Time: 10 minutes**

**Cook Time: 8-10 minutes to fry, or 15-20 minutes to bake**

Ingredients:

- 3 firm avocados, skin and stone removed, cut into ½ inch/1cm thick slices (or slightly thicker if you prefer)
- 4oz/115g almond flour
- 3oz/85g dried parmesan
- 2 tsp ground black pepper
- Olive oil if frying
- Mayonnaise for dipping

**Method:**

1.  If you are going to bake them, heat oven to 350°F/180°C/Gas mark 4.

2.  Take two small bowls, and pour in the almond flour into one. In the other, mix the dried parmesan with the pepper (if you like spicy, you could use paprika or cayenne instead – bit of a kick!)

3.  Dip the avocado slices first into the flour and then into the parmesan mix.

4.  To fry, heat olive oil over a medium heat, and carefully place the slices of avocado into the pan. Cook on both sides for 4-5 minutes, watching carefully to see they don't burn.

5.  If baking, place on a lined baking tray and cook for 10 minutes, turn over and cook the other side for a further 5 – 8 minutes.

Meltingly yummy!!

| Nutritional Value | per Portion (6 pieces) |
|---|---|
| Calories | 210 |
| Fat | 18.5g |
| Carbs | 9.8g |
| Protein | 3.2g |

# Keto Brunch Burger

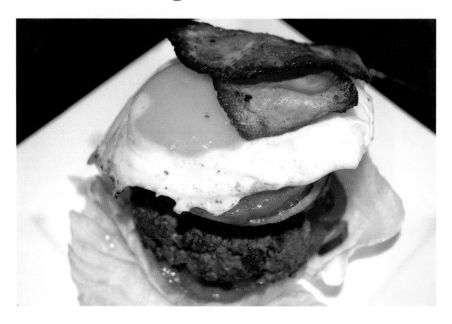

This is a great burger for breakfast, brunch, lunch or dinner. As long as you don't use burger buns, this dish is relatively low in carbohydrates, but with sufficient protein and fat for this diet. Use any amount of salad items to fill you up as these carry little or no carbs.

**Serves: 4**

**Preparation Time: 15 minutes**

**Cook Time: 10-15 minutes**

Ingredients:

- 1lb/450g ground beef
- 2 tomatoes, sliced into 8 rings
- 4 lettuce leaves, or more
- 8 red onion rings
- 2 tsp strong mustard
- 2 cloves garlic, crushed or minced
- 4 pieces bacon

- 4 eggs
- Ground black pepper
- 2 tbsp olive oil/butter

**Method:**

1. In a large bowl, mix together the ground beef, mustard and garlic. Season with pepper. Shape into burger patties.

2. Grill the bacon and when just crisp, remove and keep warm.

3. In a skillet or frying pan, fry the burgers over a low to medium heat for 4 minutes on one side. Flip over, and cook for 4 minutes on the other side. Test the middle – if the blood still runs, cook for a further 2 minutes on each side.

4. Crack the 4 eggs into a separate pan and gently fry in a little olive oil or butter.

5. While the eggs are frying, take 4 plates and place a lettuce leaf and a tomato ring on each. Place a burger on to each, and top with the onion rings, and another tomato ring.

6. Place the fried egg and a piece of bacon on the top of each burger.

7. Serve.

This recipe is great with avocado fries or coleslaw (see recipes) but remember to add the nutritional values on to this recipe.

| Nutritional Value | per Burger (no side dishes) |
|---|---|
| Calories | 407 |
| Fat | 30.5g |
| Carbs | Under 1g (trace) |
| Protein | 28.5g |

# Treat Yourself Coconut Sponge Pudding

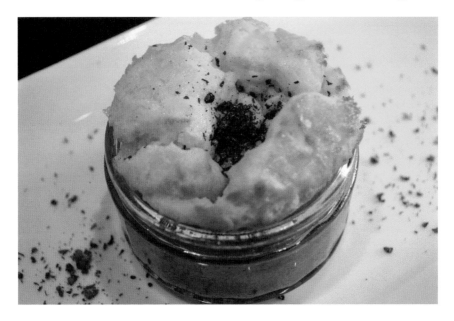

So delicious, so easy to make so enjoy! These look quite spectacular as they rise and resemble soufflés – very impressive!

**Serves: 4**

**Preparation Time: Less than 10 minutes**

**Cook Time: 15 minutes**

Ingredients:

- 3oz/85g coconut flour
- 2 eggs
- 2oz/55g granulated sugar substitute
- 2oz/55g coconut flakes
- 1 tsp baking powder
- 4 tbsp heavy cream
- ½ tsp vanilla essence
- 1oz/30g dark chocolate, grated

- 1 tbsp butter
- ½ tbsp butter for greasing

## Method:

1. Lightly grease 4 ramekin dishes. Heat oven to 180°C/350°F/Gas mark 4.

2. Cream the butter and sugar substitute together. Add the eggs and mix together gently, to avoid curdling.

3. Add the coconut flour, vanilla essence and baking powder, mix well to form a 'dropping' mixture.

4. Pour or spoon into greased dishes. Bake in the oven for 15 minutes.

5. Remove from the oven, and serve hot, with the grated chocolate over the top.

| Nutritional Value | per Portion |
|-------------------|-------------|
| Calories | 171 |
| Fat | 17.8g |
| Carbs | 4.2g |
| Protein | 3.7g |

# Spiced Salmon with Stir Fried Greens

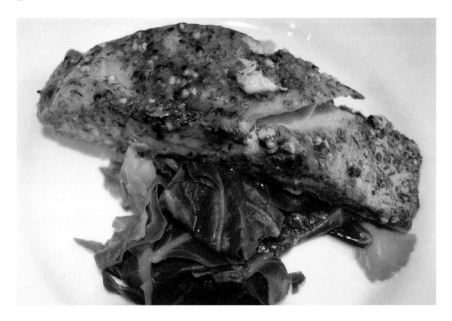

Salmon is the 'king of the sea' or freshwater royalty! Lightly spiced and roasted, it is tender and melts in the mouth. Full of Omega 3 properties, it is always a wonderful addition to any diet.

**Serves: 4**

**Preparation Time: Less than 10 minutes**

**Cook Time: 15 minutes or less**

Ingredients:

- 4 x 5oz/140g boneless salmon fillets
- 2 tbsp olive oil
- 1 tbsp fresh coriander, finely chopped
- Juice of 2 limes, plus grated rind
- 1 tsp ground black pepper or ground mixed pepper
- 1inch/2cm piece of lemongrass

- 1½lbs/675g mixed greens, such as cabbage, spinach, kale or broccoli
- 2 cloves of garlic, finely chopped
- Extra olive oil for frying greens

Method:

1. Heat oven to 350°F/180°C/Gas mark 4.

2. Prepare the marinade for the salmon by grinding the coriander and lemongrass to a paste, using the olive oil and lime juice and rind. Season with ground pepper.

3. Marinate the salmon fillets in the mix for 10 minutes or longer if you can.

4. On a lined and lightly oiled baking tray, place the salmon fillets and pour over the marinade evenly on each fillet. Place in the oven and bake for 15 minutes, checking after 10 minutes to ensure that the fillets are not overcooking.

5. Whilst the fillets are cooking, roughly chop all your greens. Place the oil in the frying pan over a medium heat, add the chopped garlic and fry until soft. Add the green and stir fry for 6-8 minutes until al dente.

6. Remove the salmon from the oven, and serve on top of a portion of the fried greens.

| Nutritional Value | per Portion |
|---|---|
| Calories | 312 |
| Fat | 21.7g |
| Carbs | 6.5g |
| Protein | 22.4g |

# Day 7

# Scotch Eggs Keto Style

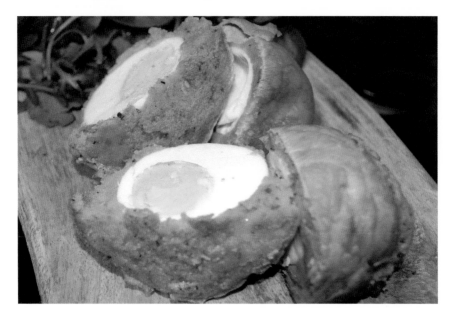

There are many 'bland' scotch eggs sold in supermarkets these days, and there is nothing more delicious than making your own from scratch. No high carb coatings of breadcrumbs, pure and simple seasoned sausage meat, wrapped with bacon – couldn't be better!

**Serves: 4**

**Preparation Time: 20 minutes**

**Cook Time: 20-25 minutes (including boiling eggs)**

Ingredients:

- 1lb/450g good quality sausage meat
- 4 eggs
- 4 strips of bacon
- Handful of parsley, finely chopped
- Ground black pepper to taste
- 2 tsp onion powder

Method:

1.  Heat oven to 350°F/180°C/Gas mark 4

2.  Hard boil the eggs for approximately 7 minutes. Cool and peel.

3.  Place the sausage meat in a bowl; add the onion powder and parsley, mix thoroughly together. Season with ground black pepper to taste.

4.  Portion the meat mix into four, and make a round of each portion. Place egg in the middle and wrap with the sausage meat. Wrap a slice of bacon around each, and secure with a cocktail stick.

5.  Line a baking tray with foil, place the scotch eggs on to the tray and bake in the oven for about 15 minutes, until the sausage meat is cooked and the bacon is crisp.

6.  Serve with a little watercress garnish.

| Nutritional Value | per Portion |
|---|---|
| Calories | 334 |
| Fat | 23.8g |
| Carbs | 1.4g |
| Protein | 27.8g |

# Ham and Prawn Roulades

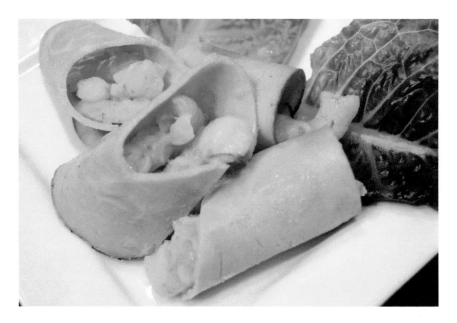

Easy to make, fresh prawns are better, but frozen will do, squeezed of any excess water.

**Serves: 4 (2 roulades each)**

**Preparation Time: 10 minutes**

**Cook Time: No cooking required**

Ingredients:

- 8 slices of deli ham (approximately 8oz/225g)
- 6oz/170g small prawns (cooked) or shrimp cut into pieces
- 3 tbsp mayonnaise
- 1 tbsp low sugar ketchup
- Freshly ground black pepper
- Juice of half lemon, squeezed and no pips

Method:

1. In a small bowl, mix together the mayonnaise, ketchup, lemon and black pepper to taste.

2. Put in the prawns/shrimp, mix thoroughly.

3. Lay out the ham slices, and place the mixture, divided evenly on to each piece of ham, to one side.

4. Roll up the ham so that all the mixture is enclosed. Cut each roulade in half if necessary.

5. Serve.

| Nutritional Value | per Portion |
|---|---|
| Calories | 173 |
| Fat | 7.8g |
| Carbs | 2.75g |
| Protein | 24.5g |

# Cauliflower and Chorizo Cheese

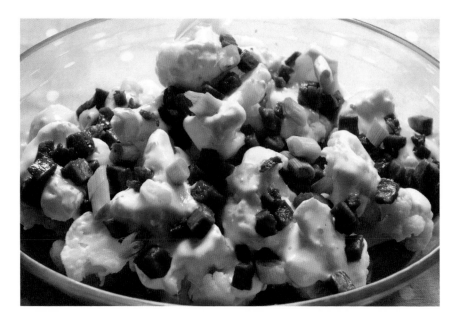

Just like a normal cauliflower cheese, but with the addition to little cubes of spicy chorizo to give it more flavor and a little more interest for a lunchtime meal.

**Serves: 4**

**Preparation Time: 10 minutes**

**Cook Time: 20 minutes**

Ingredients:

- 1½lb/675g cauliflower, broken into florets
- 6oz/170g chorizo, cubed
- 8oz/225g cheddar, grated
- 8oz/225g heavy cream
- 2 heaped tsp strong yellow mustard
- Pepper to taste

Method:

1.  Heat oven to 350°F/180°C/Gas mark 4.

2.  Bring a large pan of water to the boil and pop in the cauliflower florets. Cook for approximately 10-15 minutes until tender, but not mushy.

3.  Whilst the cauliflower is cooking, fry off the chorizo (no oil needed, as the chorizo creates its own oil). Leave to one side.

4.  In a smaller pan, gently heat the cream. Stir in the mustard and cheese until melted. Scatter over the chorizo cubes.

5.  Place in a baking dish and pop into the oven for about 10 minutes, until warmed through and just bubbling.

6.  Season with pepper and serve.

| Nutritional Value | per Portion |
|---|---|
| Calories | 670 |
| Fat | 57g |
| Carbs | 5g |
| Protein | 30g |

# Chocolate Brownie Tray Bake

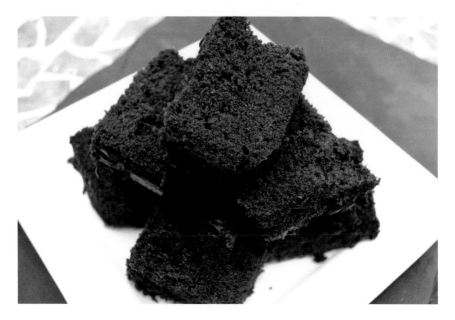

Tasty morning coffee or afternoon tea snack with some healthy chia seeds to provide you with extra Omega 3. This recipe could also be served as a dessert if required, and is useful for lunchboxes.

**Serves: 12 pieces**

**Preparation Time: 15 minutes**

**Cook Time: 40-45 minutes**

Ingredients:

- 4oz/115g butter, melted
- 2oz/55g coconut flour
- 2oz/55g ground flaxseed or flaxseed meal
- 5oz/140g unsweetened cocoa powder
- 6oz/170g granulated sugar substitute
- 3oz/85g soft cream cheese
- 4fl.oz/120ml water (more if required)

- 4 large eggs
- 1 tbsp chia seeds
- 2 tsp vanilla extract
- 1 tsp baking soda

Method:

1. Chia seeds need to be soaked with water before using, so that they form a sticky gel. Soak for approximately 20 minutes.

2. Lightly grease an 8 x 8 inch/20 x 20cm baking tin. Heat oven to 325°F/160°C/Gas mark 3.

3. Once the gel has formed, take a large bowl and mix the gel in with the flour and ground flax seed, and then whisk in the eggs.

4. Gently mix all the other ingredients into the bowl, whisk to prevent any lumps, but do not beat. Pour the cake mix into the prepared tin. Leave to one side.

5. In a small pan, very gently warm the cream cheese until slightly runny, and then swirl the cheese into the batter mixture.

6. Place in the oven and bake for 40-45 minutes, until a skewer inserted into the middle of the brownie mix comes out clean, and the top of the mix is firm to the touch.

| Nutritional Value | per Piece |
|---|---|
| Calories | 180 |
| Fat | 15.7g |
| Carbs | 6.6g |
| Protein | 5.9g |

# Oriental Sea Bass Parcels

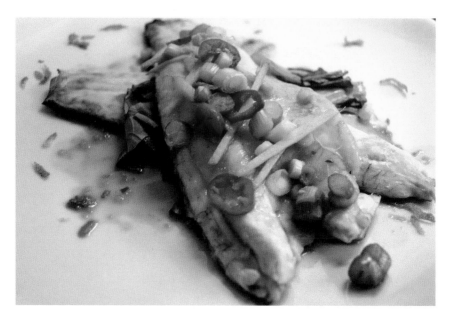

Sea bass is a delicious fish, with a very delicate taste that can take most sauces. It pairs perfectly with hints of Chinese or Thai spices and is very quick to cook and prepare. You can substitute sea bass for other white fish fillets, such as cod, haddock or similar, but adjust cooking times as these can tend to be a 'fatter' fish' and will need longer to cook.

**Serves: 4**

**Preparation Time: 15 minutes**

**Cook Time: 15 minutes**

Ingredients:

- 4 sea bass fillets
- 2 pak choi (bok choi), thickly sliced
- 4 scallions/spring onions, finely chopped
- 1 small red chilli, finely chopped
- 2 cm/ ¾ inch fresh ginger, cut into thin matchsticks (if you don't like ginger, you can use something like carrots or radish)

- 4 tbsp sweet chilli sauce
- Juice of 1 lime, plus grated zest

Method:

1. Heat oven to 200 C/380 F/Gas Mark 6.

2. Mix together the sweet chilli sauce, juice of the lime and set aside.

3. Take 4 large square pieces of foil and place the pak choi slices in the centre of each. Place the sea bass on top of the pak choi.

4. Scatter the scallions, ginger, lime zest and chilli over each piece. Top with a little of the sweet chilli dressing.

5. Fold over the foil to form a package, sealing at both ends so that the steam does not escape. Cook for 10 -15 minutes in the oven, depending how thick the fillets are.

6. Open the packages and remove each fillet on to a plate. Top with a little more of the dressing.

7. Serve with an Oriental salad of pak choi, radishes, diced cucumber or stir fried greens.

| Nutritional Value | per Portion |
|---|---|
| Calories | 137 |
| Fat | 2g |
| Carbs | 11g |
| Protein | 18g |

# Thank You!

Thank you for purchasing this meal plan book. If you found it useful, please take a moment to leave a review.

As a gift for purchasing this book, you can get the bonus recipe, free printable meal plan and shopping list by visiting the link below:

http://gotorecipecookbooks.com/ketogenic-diet-1/

If you enjoyed this book, collect the entire set:

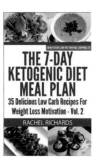

http://www.amazon.com/dp/B00KLDHDWO

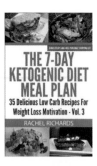

http://www.amazon.com/dp/B00NJD8UVG

The box set is also available:

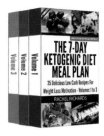

http://www.amazon.com/dp/B00OK14B4Q

You might also like this other book by the same author:

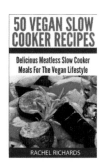

http://www.amazon.com/dp/B00LODQ9T8

To stay updated on the latest recipe books by Rachel Richards, please visit the website at:

http://RachelRichardsRecipeBooks.com

Until next time.

Rachel Richards

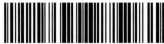

Printed in Great Britain
by Amazon